Does

Reiki

Love

Heal

Cancer?

Transcribed

True Stories of Spiritual Healing

Rev. Mike Wanner

Table of Contents

Does Reiki Love Heal Cancer?

Transcribed

True Stories of Spiritual Healing

Introduction

Hello, this is Mike Wanner

And I have some stories to tell you.

Do you like love stories?

Let me tell you Mickey's story. A love story about one loving sister who wanted to deal with the traumatic news about her sister's cancer. This story is about what one can do to help. The story shows that there's always something that one can do.

It's about one's own power to choose a positive approach regardless of what happens to you or those that you love.

The shocking news turned into a success story.

The success of this family is about living through it together. With the support that came from this union, they collectively affirm the power of their love behind the a willingness to thrive in the face of adversity. They grew closer together and the family blossomed from a point of desperation.

May each of you who hear these words remember always that when bad things threaten, there are only two things to focus upon. You can stay in fear and attract more fear into your life because what you focus on increases in your life or you can move forward with love and attract more love into your life because what you focus on increases in your life.

You always get to choose what you attract. You always have a choice. Acknowledging your responsibility and power to choose is awesomely significant in your ability to handle any situation, and to help heal yourself.

Too many people place all the responsibility on the doctors and the nurses. In this country, we are blessed with magnificent medical resources and then, we undermine our capability by not doing our part.

We are each of us in a package, which includes the body, the mind and the spirit. The medical professionals deal with the body issues and take notice of the mind and spirit as they impact on the clinical aspects.

The more that we can do to work on our mind and spirit, the bigger opportunity the medical professionals have to reach the pinnacle of medical success for us.

Now, I want to move into the story.

As we go forward, please look for the ideas that come into your head as your path to follow.

This story is about this family. Even if you don't have a family, you can choose an aggressive positive loving path to help yourself and others.

There's an old saying that if you want to have a friend, be one. This is great advice Because when you focus on others, they feel better and so do you.

If you have been drawn to this message, know that you have significant power to influence your physical condition, your life and the lives of countless others.

The story starts in Philadelphia, Pennsylvania.

I live here. The story is about a friend of mine from Toastmasters and her family.

My friend's name is Rosemary but we call her Mickey.

She has heard me speak about healthcare many times and more recently, she has heard me talk about the power of the mind in our healing and also complementary methods of healthcare, such as energy healing.

She was always interested in what I was saying but she had a real life to deal with, just like the rest of us.

When she called me on a Monday evening, her telephone message sounded desperate. I returned her call and we kept messaging one another.

We finally talked on Tuesday morning and she was beside herself with fear. Her sister wanted to meet me right away.

It seems that Mickey had been talking about my speeches and now that her sister was faced with a crisis, I was on the mind.

The crisis was her sister had cancer surgery on Monday and was advised that she needed more surgery and radiation, and chemotherapy.

This was the last news that this family wanted to hear. They had lost their mother to the disease in a very unpleasant passing.

The sister was been watched medically for symptoms so that a repeat could be avoided and then, here they were.

I agreed to meet Joan on Thursday and I offered her an Integrated Energy Therapy session to relieve some of her suppressed feelings. Joan's mood changed dramatically within the session.

The main on-going support that was to be offered was to empower the family to help Joan heal.

We scheduled a private Reiki course for Mickey, Joan, Joan's sister Peg and Joan's sister in law Terry.

The class would be two days later, Mothers' Day weekend. The class would empower them all to provide Reiki to Joan.

I refer to Reiki as God's greatest gift.

It is so simple that youngsters can learn it.

A friend of mine has a Holistic Centre in Wycombe, Bucks County and they teach a Magic Hands course there, just for the kids.

Can you imagine a grandparent receiving Reiki from their little grandchild with hot Reiki hands. While hot Reiki hands are a symbol for many of the healing but Reiki works whether hands get hot or not,

Whether the practitioner or recipient felt heat, or not.

Reiki works as long as the practitioner has been attuned by a master and the recipient is willing at some level to receive.

Reiki is at the first level basically, a hands-on healing modality where the practitioner lays hands on or slightly over the recipient. The practitioner channels universal life force, universal energy to a willing recipient.

The energy helps the recipient come to a more natural balance where the most powerful healing system for that recipient, their own body, will start to do the natural job that the body was designed to do and this enhances any medical intervention. It helps to speed the healing.

Reiki is a spiritual process where the Divine is contacted to provide the source energy for the recipient. The effect is spiritual and individual.

There is not a religious affiliation. Reiki works for the believers of all religions. The Divine orchestration of the special course for Joan became apparent on Friday morning about 7:30 am. My guidance kicked in and reminded me of a lady that I had met at an Introduction to Reiki being conducted by one of my students the prior Sunday at an Episcopal Church.

The lady was attached to an oxygen bottle so that she could go to church and pray for a lung transplant.

My guidance was that this lady was at least as deserving as Joan and why shouldn't she be included in the class.

I took the guidance and called my student, who called the pastor and got the phone number and called the lady. The lady called me on Friday night and was thrilled with the idea. She wanted to know when did I get this idea? I told her about 7:30 Friday morning.

She told me that was the time she told God that she didn't care anymore. She was giving up and she didn't care what happens. Her name is Nancy. She joined us for what proved to be an unforgettable weekend.

Now, We get to Mickey and the conversation we had about the class.

Conversation with Mickey

Mike-

Hello Mickey!

I'm ready to record your story.

Are you ready for my questions?

Mickey-

Yes, hi Mike!

Mike-

Hi!

Okay Mickey

Tell me the background story behind everything that happened. Tell me first about your mother, then about the precautionary watch on Joan.

Mickey-

Okay Mike

In my mother's situation, my mother passed away in 1993 from breast cancer.

She didn't let us know that she had breast cancer.

She never went for check-ups or anything until she was almost at end stage.

So it was a particularly tough death.

And I think from that point on, my sister Peg, my sister Joan and I, and my sister in law Theresa, to a certain extent, were always worried who would be the hereditary one to develop breast cancer.

In March, my sister went to the doctor for mammography.

Now, they have been watching her very closely since my mother's death because she had calcifications in her breasts but they were no lumps and there was nothing to suggest that there was a problem at that point.

However, three radiologists from _____ read that X-ray in April and said that she wanted her to go in and have further testing done. She went to the doctor by herself because they really didn't think there was a problem.

And even the doctor assured her that she didn't think that anything was wrong but they would go ahead with a needle biopsy, just to be on the safe side.

So, really, our family wasn't that concerned because the doctors didn't seem that concerned.

When Joan went into the needle biopsy, my brother and my sister Peg and I went with her and her son John and we waited in the waiting room and the doctor came out and said everything went fine.

But my sister, Peg, cautioned me that meant everything about the needle biopsy went fine, not necessarily the results but we still went with the idea that the doctor had said that she didn't think that there was anything wrong and Joan went for the results of that needle biopsy by herself.

And I got a call at work from Joan, saying that she had breast cancer and she was going to have a mastectomy. It was like the whole scene of my mother's death just flashed before my eyes.

And I panicked and I was just a ball of fear.

And I really didn't know how to handle it.

I couldn't even handle it.

I just couldn't even handle it

And my first instinct was, just to run away from it.

I didn't feel as though I could be any support for Joan because I was just totally remembering about my mother and I was sure in my mind that this is going to be the end result for Joan.

And pretty selfishly, I didn't feel as though I could go through what we went through with my mother again.

But since it is my sister, I knew that I would have to go through it but the way I was going to go through it was really, in my mind, not a very supportive way.

So, I spent the week after I got the news, just grieving, just crying every single day. I remembered that I had to work while my mother was sick and I guess I went a little bit crazy in a way.

I went into work and I was hysterical and I just said to my boss, lay me off because I just can't work. I'm going to take care of my sister.

And meanwhile, my sister was going to work every day and she was upset by the news but I was totally hysterical all the time. And it was a complete panic hopeless experience state and my mind just would not let me get rid of the former picture of my mother.

I was just really petrified. I knew that I couldn't remain in this high state of anxiety but I really didn't know what to do about it but all the time I remembered about you. And you had done an integrated energy session on me and I remembered how good I felt then but I still didn't feel as though any of the energy work can help us here.

I was convinced that my sister was going to go down the same path as my mother. But I did call you.

Thank God and in that conversation, I got a sense that maybe there was something I could do to make a difference.

And I had mentioned to Joan about the session that you and I had with the Integrated Energy and with all the chaos and confusion, and crying, and caring on and all that effort I didn't mention it to her anymore.

And she, one night, said to me, I would like to meet Mike and have the integrated energy. And I will never really forget that night Mike because when she came in, she just looked older. She's only 46 years old, which I forgot to mention.

Mike-

Was that the night of the surgery?

14

Mickey-

No, that was after the needle biopsy surgery.

.

That was after the needle biopsy because she was still sore.

I think that's a day after the needle biopsy.

But before...I'm getting confused with the time

So much happening in a month's time.

It gets a little bit confused in my mind But I know she has had surgery. She had either already had a mastectomy or just the needle biopsy when she had the integrated energy. But I just remembered the difference.

Mike-

Well, the integrated energy she had, the Thursday after the biopsy.

Mickey-

Okay, thanks for clearing it up for me.

Because it's kind of, like, a blurr. What I remember is...

Mike-

That's when they told her that she had to have another surgery and she had to have chemo.

Mickey-

Oh, right

Mike-

And that's when things crashed.

Mickey-

Then, they really crashed.

That's right.

Because when they did the original mastectomy, that was another bit of bad news for her because they thought that she would just have that Mastectomy, have the reconstruction, and be able to, perhaps, to take a drug, like, Tamoxifen or something, to prevent a problem in the future.

However, another surprise for the doctor was that when they removed the breast and sent it to pathology, they found the second cancer, which was invasive.

The first cancer was in the duct and the calcifications but the second cancer was invasive.

It had invaded the breast tissue around it and was a deadly form of cancer that would probably have killed her. It would not have shown up on mammography for at least another year. So, now, she's facing a second cancer. I mean a second test.

Mike-

Yes, but there's a blessing in here also

Mickey-

Yes, the blessing is that without the mastectomy, they would never have found it.

Mike-

Right

Mickey-

And you kept telling me to search for the blessing in all that's going on and I just couldn't see it.

I was still in that well of hopelessness.

But you certainly helped Joan too because that night, because I saw her come in one way and go out another with the integrated energy but during our conversation, you mentioned the Reiki.

And I always know that I get a really great feeling when you could do the energy treatment on me or even when we have a conversation and sooner or later, you can pull me down from the ceiling and possibly see a blessing.

Mike-

But I only did one session on you.

Mickey-

I know, I know but that was enough, that was enough. It's like steering the Titanic around.

Because I really, I mean you knew because you said to me on the phone that night – You could hear the fear in my voice.

Mike-

I did a little light work with you on the phone.

Mickey-

Oh, okay

Mike-

And that gave you some relief.

But I mean, the only actual.

Well I think I did that twice.

Mickey-

Right.

Mike-

But the only actual session I had with you was the integrated energy session.

Mickey-

But you could clearly hear the panic in my voice that night.

You told me that it was because of me too, not just Joan.

Because, you know, sometimes with cancer, we tend do think just of the person who has the cancer.

But actually, it's just such a family disease that it affects everybody.

And with fear and I think the normal reaction is fear for that loved one

Mike-

But, you know, fear is a prayer for something that you don't want.

So, when you're in fear and you're stuck in that fear of that situation, you are energetically attracting that, which you don't want.

Mickey-

Right.

And every time you would say that to me.

Mike-

The law of attraction.

One of the universal laws.

Mickey-

And when you would say that to me, then..I just didn't know how to stop my mind.

Really.

I really didn't know how to get control.

But each time I talk to you or saw you, I did feel that I was gaining a little bit but it wasn't until that weekend when we did the Reiki attunements that, I really came out of that hole. It was, like, a transformation.

And it was just such a wonderful, wonderful thing.

But anyway, I'm getting a little ahead of myself.

So you suggested that maybe we do learn Reiki in order to help myself and my sister and would my family members, who were supporting Joan when she went to Chemotherapy also want to learn?

We did not want to be people that just sat and hold her hand during chemotherapy.

I wanted to be more of a support but I knew that I needed some other modality of operating to be able to do that.

So, I took a risk and I called my sister, Peg, and my sister in law, Terry and asked them if they want to learn Reiki so that we could be a support system for Joan.

You kept telling me that instead of sitting around and saying, the house is on fire, the house is on fire, we could literally get to put our hands on her and have something happen.

More powerful than just saying, oh my God, isn't this awful,

Mike-

Yeah, it's the elimination of helplessness.

Mickey-

so...

Mike-

Which also eliminates the panic and the fear, and the hopelessness, and all that other stuff.

Mickey-

And I'll tell you Mike, I really, I wanted to believe you. I wanted to believe you but I really had my doubts that anything could take this terror away from me.

Now, my sister was the one with the cancer.

I was the one with the terror even more than her.

And when she went in for the lymph node surgery, Thank God the lymph nodes were clear. The bone scan was clear also and I started to see things a little better about the physical end.

And of course, with each thing going from all bad news to starting to get some good news, Joan herself was starting to feel a little bit more powerful but you could really see the effects of getting one bad piece of news after another.

Because Joan at that point, before the regular treatment, We would go to the doctors with her and she would never say a word and as soon as the doctor would start to speak, you could see her physically start to shake. Her legs would jump up and down under the table and she would just, her whole demeanor was very passive and just frightened.

And most of the time, she would not remember what the doctor said so, it became...my brother, Bill or my sister, Peg, or my job to listen.

Mike-

Sure is was bad news that she didn't want to hear, so she would block it out.

Mickey-

Right

So, we would have to tell her actually what happened at the doctor's because she just was numbed out and not there.

So, when you said that you would be willing to give us the Reiki attunements, I took it upon myself to call my family and they just jumped on the opportunity because we love Joan and we wanted to support her in a powerful way.

And from our conversation, I just start to get a sense that this is something that we all needed to learn and to be able to do. Not just for Joan but for ourselves. From what you told me, we could do it. Reiki ourselves and that would bring healing and calmness, and peace to us.

Mike-

And did it?

Mickey-

Of course it did, of course it did. I am no longer a doubting Thomas. I don't have to be overcome by doubt. It's been proven over and over with me in my own life as well as with Joan.

So, we met that weekend and you brought Nancy who is a dear lovely person and she just fit right in with our group.

And it wasn't all serious stuff, we had a lot of laughter over the weekend. The attunement was so serious and I was so moved by the attunement and by your generosity in helping me and my family. I remember, I think it was the second attunement, the tears were just running down my face because I just was starting to get the peace and the power of Reiki.

And we all loved it. We all loved it.

And the difference is so hard to describe, the difference.

Mike-

But there's a difference between you all. The interrelationship between you all was different on Sunday than it was on Saturday.

Mickey-

Oh yes. Right, the shared experience.

The shared experience in the heartfelt wanting to get this and to have this for our family, really bonded us together. I don't think Peg and Joan, and Terry and I have spent that many hours together in years. Because we all lead busy lives and we all have our own problems and we all have our own children and families. It was just nice. It was just nice to share that with them. And to be able to have that (Reiki) available to me anytime I wanted it to. The weekend was just beautiful.

After everybody left on Sunday, I was just sitting in this chair and I'm thinking something is different, something is different. I feel different than I did on Friday. I feel different on the whole idea of Cancer. I feel different about what I'm able to offer my sister. And the amazing part is that Joan felt different about her own Cancer and her relationship to me and Terry, and Peg. It was just evident. We just really enjoyed that weekend in getting the Reiki attunement.

And shortly after that, Joan was to start chemotherapy.

Mike-

So?

Mickey-

And me, the coward of the county and the person who needs to go to Oz for courage said I'll go with you to the chemotherapy. And that itself, is what I call a miraculous transformation because if anybody would have told me that I would be hanging out at the Cancer Center, I would have said, no way, not in my wildest dreams.

And it has been an experience for me, a change in me that just will last my lifetime.

So, Joan and I went off to Temple's Cancer Center and an amazing thing happened. She was hooked up to the chemotherapy and she would be standing with the intravenous drip going in her arm and giving me Reiki.

Mike-

Great

Mickey-

And then, we would change positions.

And some of the doctors and nurses would go by and they would look at us rather strangely because where a lot of the other people were just in there getting their treatments, you would hear a lot of laughter coming from me and Joan.

We would be present and it wasn't a big, horrible serious process.

Mike-

Right, you were enjoying the life you have.

Mickey-

Right.

And we talked about my daughter's upcoming wedding and what she was going to wear. And I started to really be awed by the change in her.

For instance, they told her that she would lose her hair in the first treatment. And to me, that was a particular mind blower because when my mother was sick, that was the one thing that always made me cry was the hair loss.

But I found myself saying Joan, you know, if it were me, I can't tell you what to do. I think I would just cut it off right now and have a choice in the matter. And then, the following Sunday morning she called me and she said, "well I did it, I cut my hair off."

And my brother took her to get two beautiful wigs and she just was joking about things. She was doing guided imagery tapes. She was doing Reiki herself. We would go to chemotherapy and I would just be quiet. She would start in each position and get calmed down.

And then it was just a different experience. They would tell her that she would have all kinds of side effects from chemotherapy. The first treatment she did get pretty sick but that's because they didn't give her the thirty anti-nausea medicine but her symptoms or side effects or whatever you want to call it from chemotherapy have really not been that bad. They have been minimal and I do believe it's because of the Reiki.

And the laughter and the taking it from this huge life threatening, serious, horrible thing and make it manageable in her own head.

Mike-

Right. The support of the family and the support of Reiki are so powerful. They just go hand in hand to help the body relax and when the body relaxes, it can do its job of healing. The body is a beautifully designed healing machine and if you allow the body to heal by getting all the stress, the anxiety, the fear, and all the negativity out of the way, it will bring the body into balance. And automatically shift into healing mode where it does everything that it can to help the body heal itself.

The doctors and nurses are still needed. It's just, like, if you have a bonfire and you wanted to control it. You could choose to put more wood on the fire or take some off. You know, you're better off taking wood off the fire.

When you laugh, it takes wood off the fire. When you do Reiki, it takes wood off the fire. So, every time you do the quality of life things, you bring the body more into balance.

Mickey-

Well, it's been an amazing process and not only did my family bond that weekend, it continued and Joan is amazing. She did the Run for the Cure, right after her Lymph Node surgery, she did the Cancer Race for the Cure.

Mike-

How long is that?

Mickey-

The Race for the Cure, I believe, there's one on Mothers' Day, she walked it. She walked in the Survivors Walk but that was only a week after one of her surgeries.

Then there's a huge...I believe it's called The Race for the Cure, where you walk around St. Joes' University track and you get supporters. Well, people were giving her money at work supporting her and she came after that and we were all there and she had surgery a couple of days before that. She had just gotten out of the hospital and she still had drains adhesive taped to her side and walked that track several times. I mean, I would just stand there with my mouth opened.

The real transformation is in her. Now when we get to the doctors, there is no more, leg shaking, body shaking, curling in a ball of fear. Joan is there saying "let me tell you how it's going to go from now on" and it's coming from her. And I'm just there, like, wow, this is amazing. So many amazing things have happened. She got a new job at _____, she had applied for a new job right before she found out she had breast cancer and she got that division. And now, she moved up already to a secretary to a vice president there.

The social worker at the Cancer Center wants her to start a Cancer Survivor Group on campus because there are lots of people with Cancer who work there.

And I think that's the biggest thing. I'm seeing Cancer in a different way. I only saw Cancer through the filter of my mother's sickness and death when it was too late to do anything.

I think with the Reiki opening my eyes and calming me down enough to observe a little better. I'm starting to see a lot of people and it's a shame because I really wish they would find a cure for it.

I don't want to make light of all of this because it is a devastating thing to go through but I'm starting to see that you can have a life even with this diagnosis.

And it's more powerful if you have Reiki and healing energy to go along with the medical end of it. Because our doctors have been wonderful and they really didn't do anything wrong with the diagnosis.

Everything was a big surprise every time they had to tell Joan to come back in for another surgery. The visiting nurses said, there have never seen that level of healing in all those, in three or four surgeries that she had in a month time in any other of their patients.

She didn't have the pain that she's supposed to have. The doctor said she probably would need physical therapy on her arm where the Mastectomy took place. Within a week and a half to two weeks, she was able to raise her arm above her head without any pain to have them examine her. She has had the worst surgery of all. She had the Mastectomy, the reconstructions, the Lymph node surgery. She said the worst was to put the port in her arm. That is what she had the most pain from.

Maybe everything would have turned out like that but I don't think so, They physical end of it, the doctors were taking care of but I do believe that the healing and her attitude, my attitude, my sister's and brother's attitude, all changed that weekend that we got the Reiki attunement. That made the difference.

Mike-

I agree because you came together as a family behind her and she knew it. It was real. That's very important. You know, I've been doing ambulance work in this city for 30 years, and I can't tell you how many Cancer patients I've had over the years. The ones that do well in my view and this is not scientific. This is my observation. The ones that do well are the ones that have family support. When family support is there and the proper attitude is there, they can do well. And the more support they get, the better off they do.

Mickey-

That's why there should be some kind of patient support Reiki people in the Cancer Centers.

Mike-

Some Cancer Centers have that and it's something that's coming in hospitals. But it's just not quite there yet, it's very difficult to put these programs together because funding for traditional methods of care are being squeezed in these economic times.

And new programs and new ideas are not what people are looking for right now.

Mickey-

It always amazes me because I have been using Reiki now, of course, every day in my own life and I've had other experiences that if somebody told me about it, I'd be a doubting Thomas but since it as happened to me, the little things like paper cuts closing up right before my eyes and my plants living when I always had to have artificial plants before I had Reiki because real plants would not survive.

I have a good friend who I recently used Reiki on when she cut her leg pretty bad in a fall. When I went over there for dinner, I introduced her to Reiki and I did it for about 10 minutes and I did it again before I left and she said to me, during the second time I did it that, that this is really weird " I feel, like, my leg has begun to itch".

I called the next day and she said I just want to learn more about this. I want to do it myself because my leg is really looking 100 percent better than it did yesterday.

So, I just think it's wonderful and the difference that it has made for Joan and me, and Peg, and Terry. It's just really amazing. And I'll always be grateful. I'm so glad that you're my friend.

Laughter - Mike & Mickey

Mickey-

Because I was really drowning inside, really drowning in panic. My boss was probably panicky too because I've been there 15 years. I mean, I remember that day getting that phone call from her and just, the next day, just walking in and crying, and packing everything on my desk.

And I think I was scared. I mean, I must have been pretty scary Because it is scary to see somebody who's out of control.

Mike -

You were, you were so scared . It was unbelievable

I struggled to find the right things to say to you.

Mickey-

Oh! God

And you know Mike, I often think back and you can't have any regrets but I know that not everybody does make it. Reiki is not a miracle but I often think that if we had known about this and learned it when my mom was sick, her passing would have even been different.

Mike-

Yes

Mickey-

Because we would be different and we would have handled it different.

If you wanted to see panic, you just should have seen that. The only one that wasn't panicky was my mother.

It is a huge difference with Joan now. A huge difference. She's working every day. Today, she went for her last chemotherapy treatment and now she starts radiation for one month.

And she's back on her job and the amazing part is.

Mike-

Back on her new job?

Mickey-

Back on her new job. The amazing part is that she's physically could have probably went back to work two weeks after her Mastectomy. She is really doing so well, I can't believe it and she's happy.

You know, she's very positive. And whenever I sit in the chair when they give her the chemotherapy and I just watch her start her procedure before the drip and I know she's going, she starts putting her hands on the first position on the top of her head and just going through the motions.

One time a nurse came in to me one time we were there, I think it was her second treatment, and she said, "is everything alright? Because I noticed that you were standing and holding your sister on the shoulders"

And Joan and I just started laughing. And we said, yea, we're Reiki people.

And the nurse, keeps asking her questions.

Did you get that metallic taste in your mouth?

(It's common in chemotherapy)

No.

Have you had much nausea after the first bout?

No.

Have you had this, have you had that?

No. No.

She did get ulcers from one treatment in her mouth .

But she did Reiki on her mouth and they were gone within about three days. Reiki combined with the mouth wash.

But it is a combination of the Reiki and the medical.

You know, having good doctors is important too.

Mike-

Absolutely

Reiki is not a replacement for medical care.

Reiki is a complement to a good medical care and it's a good thing to help keep people in a stress reduction mode in a tranquil setting so that they don't have these stress related illnesses or complications.

Mickey-

Oh, I forgot about one important thing that happened down there, when we were waiting for Joan to get her port opened for her treatment the first time.

I remember this woman was just lying there just looking so wiped out, not with treatment yet but just ill, lying back on her pillow and her daughter was there and you can see that they were very anxious.

Then something just moved me to walk over and I saw transformation. You're right about the healing touch by just having caring concern for another human being. I started to talk to her and asked if I could put her on my prayer list and I told her that I practice Reiki and I just took her hand and told her it would go wherever she needed it.

And when I left, she was sitting up in bed with a big smile on her face, completely transformed from the woman that I first viewed from across the room.

And her daughter was laughing And I said, hey, this is Reiki. Reiki equals laughter too, It's just a wonderful energy and I'm so happy that I knew you because I just can't imagine where we would be today in this Because I have a tendency that when I panic, life stops for me.

Mike-

Yes, I know

I've talked to you before.

Mike & Mickey

Laughing

Mickey-

Joan and I actually went to see Tarzan, Saturday, in the movies.

And she was feeling a little bit awkward, She said will we be the only adults in here?

I said so what?

I mean, we are so present to life, it's not even funny.

Mike-

That's the important thing right there. It is that you live life every day and enjoy it.

And we are all going to leave the earth plain some time. But while we're here, we should be enjoying ourselves and making the best of it.

And the support of family and the support of complementary medical processes is very, very important. And I thank you for taking the time for taking my call and share your perception of how it was.

I hope that we're able to develop this message into something that can get across to others so that many, many people can be expedited through the process to a better recovery and a quicker, less painful one.

So, that's my goal.

Mickey-

And I want to thank you for being you and I say that to you every time I talk to you.

Well that was Mickey, a wonderful person to associate with.

Now, let us talk with Joan to see what she has to say about this experience.

Conversation With Joan

Hi Joan, it's Mike!-

How are you?

Joan- Hi Mike! How are you?

Mike-Oh, I'm just fine

I just got done a little while ago, working with Mickey and moving forward with this tape project.

Joan- Okay

Mike-

And I wanted to know now what you want to say on this.

Joan-

Initially with the original decision to do the biopsy, they thought there was a 95 percent chance nothing was going to be there. That it would be benign.

Mike- Okay

Joan-

There was no lump, no mass, nothing. Just calcifications that had changed. Because of my mom's background, they wanted to do this and I agreed to it.

Somehow I felt something was wrong. I wasn't comfortable with the whole situation. I went for the needle biopsy and I knew when they did not tell me right away it was benign, that something was definitely wrong.

I went back to the doctors and they did say they found a Cancer and I immediately became hysterical because that associated me with my mother. She died from Cancer and I expected that I was going to do the same thing.

I talked to the Oncologist and made my decision to have a Mastectomy with reconstruction and he said from what they could tell, that would be the only thing I would need, no chemo, no nothing because of the type of cancer that they thought it was.

I went with that but unfortunately, I did not find out until after they did the surgery two weeks later that they had found another Cancer that was infiltrating and it was aggressive.

They felt that they had it all out but they would have to do another surgery to do a Mastectomy to find out if it had spread to my Lymph nodes and also had to do a bone scan to see if it had gone into my bones.

Like I said, I was completely hysterical.

During that time, was when Mickey suggested you and Reiki and you gave me that first Integrational.

Mike-

Integrated Energy Therapy

Joan-

Integrated Energy Therapy

I was very sore at that time because it was just after surgery but I could feel the difference afterwards with my breathing was much easier and I did not realize that I had been breathing so shallow.

And when Mickey suggested we learn how to do Reiki, I was all for it because I was determined that I was beating this. It was not taking me down like it did with my mother and I was using anything I could to win, including alternative methods of healing.

Once we started doing it, I was amazed at the difference that I could feel in myself, mainly the breathing and how relaxed I could make myself become. And I think that had a big part in how I healed because right after that is when I had the second surgery and fortunately, everything came out good with that and the bone scan. But I do Reiki all the time now and I do feel, it has made a difference in my recovery.

Besides this method of Reiki healing, the traditional methods like the chemo has helped and I am doing the radiation but I believe Reiki has helped lessen any negative effects of all of these.

And whether it was done where either I've done it for myself or Mickey has done it to me during my chemo treatments, I can see a big difference. Oh, Cancer changes your life completely. You will realize you have to live for today because tomorrow is no guarantee.

Things that you feel are important are not really all that important.

And like Mickey said, we would go to the chemo sessions and we always fortunately were in a private room up until this last session, which I wasn't. My brother went with me this last time but you can see the people in their rooms and they were together and they were very quiet in the room.

Mickey and I more or less talked non-stop. I know that's hard to believe but we talked about stuff as we did Reiki on each other during the chemo treatment. And treated it, like, it was just another occurrence that you have to get through, that it is no big deal.

And you do manage to get through it. And I do believe Reiki helped the symptoms. I'm not saying I didn't get sick. I was very sick the first time. And each time, there was an exhaustion but somehow, you pull through.

And I think that is the basis of it, it does help you. And my one friend who I used Reiki on, I knew when I asked her that she had a second degree burn on her hand, on her finger that was not healing. She did not believe in Reiki and she was my best friend so I could tell by the look on her face but she was doing it to humor me. But she also thought that I shouldn't be doing it because I was so called sick and I assured her that from the time of the surgery, I no longer consider myself as having Cancer. I consider myself as cured and everything else is just preventative.

I did the Reiki on her and she didn't say anything. The next day she called me and said she was done because it had started to heal and within two days, it was completely gone. And she called her boyfriend who was a paramedic and was telling him all about it and he said he knew all about Reiki and he believed in it too.

Now she wants me to do her daughter. She's just stunned that it works And she wants me to do her mother also who has Cancer but she is in the end stages. It's amazing.

Mike-

Yes

Well, your family doing it together was a very special thing too, I think

Joan- Oh, definitely

I could not have made this. I don't think I would have made it this far if it hadn't been for my family, my sisters and my brother, and my sister in law. You know, they have been by my side non-stop and I think that has had a whole lot to do with it.

Mike-

Yes

Well, from everything that I've heard and everything you're telling me you're doing great. And I'm so happy that the outcome is so positive.

Joan-

People tell me that I look better than I did before I had the cancer.

Mike-

The difference between what I saw on Thursday night before we did the IET session and what I saw after the Reiki class was as different as night and day and you just went on from there.

Joan-

Something just clicked with that session and then with the learning how to do Reiki, it just clicked that this is something that is going to help me and I'm not powerless with this disease.

Mike-

That's the biggie, You just said it .

You are not powerless.

See, a lot of people feel they're victimized and they have no control anymore and once they know that they have control and they can do stuff. And it's not just Reiki that they can do, everything that's related to their lifestyle can change.

Everything from their food, to their work, to the how much they sleep, to the medication and their whole life experience.

Joan-

Well, to be open to change. For the whole week, I did nothing but sleep. I was exhausted, I've never been this tired since I started taking chemo. I got to a point where I cannot actually move and it is an effort to even get a glass of water. I would feel guilty for that before but not anymore because I just say this is what my body needs. This is what it needs and what it is going to get. It is going to sleep.

Mike-

True

Joan-

There's always tomorrow

Mike-

That is marvelous.

You're listening to yourself.

You're taking care of yourself.

You're learning.

And you're growing.

And you're going.

And you're doing.

And you're living.

Joan-

This has been a gift in a strange sort of way.

Mike-

Well, for one thing I think the gift was that this invasive level of Cancer would have been devastating had it not been detected early.

Joan-

Oh, it was.

I was told that this one would have killed me .

Mike-

Right.,

Joan-

And I was very fortunate.

That had it not been my mother's history, they would not have done this in the first place. So, in a convoluted way it was a blessing.

Mike-

The blessing is always there.

You just have to find it.

You have to want to see it.

Joan-

Yes and I am sorry that I didn't do more radical and have them both done at the same time. And I know, next year I am looking at getting the other side done. But that's fine. You know, I could deal with that.

Mike-

But the amount of Reiki that you're doing and everything else you're doing, that's positive. Who knows what next year will bring.

Joan-

Oh, Who knows?

I've been thinking about that but I know I'll survive it and it's no big deal but this is not the end. You know, it took my mother but it's not taking me.

And in some way, it had pulled us apart with my mother and with me it's done the opposite and pulled us all together. It has made us realize what we have in each other.

Mike-

Yes

Joan-

And if I didn't have it, this never would have happened.

So, in effect it had a complete opposite effect.

I just, like I said, I have control over my body.

Mike-

You sure do.

Joan-

And in, like I said, instead of bringing us apart, it brought us together.

So, it can't destroy us as a family anymore.

It took my mother, it took my father but it's not taking me.

Mike-

That's great.

That is marvelous.

Joan-

And, I think the best thing I think Reiki could help a lot of people down there just by the relaxation part.

Mike-

Yes, stress reduction.

Joan-

Definitely! I noticed there's a big difference and even this last time, they put us into a common room and I was with my brother and it wasn't the same as being with Mickey because we didn't get to do the Reiki the whole day but I had my tapes from the _____ Cancer Center and I started listening to some of them and that completely made a difference.

This is not as catastrophic as you make it, you can make it as a positive experience.

Mike-

And you have.

Joan-

It would be a lot easier for me to have given up and say, okay, I am like my mother. I would have been dead in 18 months. But if I am, so what? For the 18 months, I am going to enjoy life.

Mike-

That's a great philosophy.

Joan-

You know? And the way I feel, I feel better now than I ever felt.

Mike

Good.

Well, thanks a lot.

Joan-

Oh, you're welcome.

Mike- Take care. I'll see you.

Joan- Okay. Bye. Bye.

Mike- Bye and thanks.

Well, that was Joan reviewing Mickey's Reiki interview.

Since the interview, Joan pointed out to me that Mickey and I aren't perfect because we need to get all the dates in the right sequence and we got the race titles in a little bit of disorder.

So, for clarity, she wanted me to give you the particulars about the races.

The Race for the Cure is for breast cancer survivors and it is held on Mothers' Day every year. It is sponsored by the Susan G. Komen Foundation.

The Relay for Life is for all types of Cancer survivors and it is a marathon. The sponsor is the American Cancer Society.

Introduction to the Third Interview

I recently read a marvelous case history that I wish to share with you. The practitioner studied Reiki with me and my teaching partners. She is a Japanese citizen who never heard of Reiki in Japan.

She learned about it here in America and studied it here. She has a Bachelor's Degree in nursing and is a member of the Medical Mission Sisters community. She just completed Holistic Studies here in Philadelphia and is now off to India. She is a delightful representation of God blessing us. She is Sister Yumiko Nobue.

Sister Yumiko speaks English fluently but she does not write it as well. She asked the daughter of the Cancer survivor to write the case history and she did. The daughter has also agreed to be interviewed and record this story with me.

Conversation with Dr. Pat

It is my pleasure now to introduce to you a doctor of Psychology, Doctor Pat.

Hello Pat!

How are you doing?

Dr. Pat-

I'm okay.

How are you?

Mike-

Oh, just great, just great.

We are ready for the case history now.

Would you like to tell us the background and the story about your mother?

Dr. Pat-

Thank you very much.

My mom was diagnosed with breast cancer in 1994.

She received a bilateral Lumpectomy.

So, was placed on Tamoxifen.

Now, at that time Tamoxifen was sort of a wonder drug.

People had a lot of hope, for victims of breast cancer.

Unfortunately, a side effect of Tamoxifen is Uterine cancer.

So, my mother's doctors recommended regular biopsies of the Uterus.

Her November 1997 biopsy was normal.

But the one in December of 1998 showed a stage 3 malignancy present.

Her general practitioner was unnerved by this finding since my mom had been going for months with blood tests and exams and everything had seemed normal.

And a Stage 3 malignancy is certainly not what you would expect from Tamoxifen since Tamoxifen related Cancers are usually slow moving and non-problematic and that is why they prescribe the drug.

And so, if a person would get Uterine cancer, they just perform a Hysterectomy and the problem is removed. Unfortunately, that was not the case with my mom.

They wanted to see if the Cancer had spread and get an idea of what is going on inside of her before they performed the Hysterectomy so they did a CAT scan.

And that revealed a hypodensity within the central portion of the Uterus representing the known Endometrial Neoplasm.

But there was also Ascites with infiltration of the mesentry and peritoneal wall involvement anteriorly.

And that suggested that there was a bigger problem than just the Cancer in the Cervical cavity.

The surgeon performed a full Hysterectomy at _____ Hospital on February 3rd in 1999.

He was unable to remove all the tumor from the Peritoneal wall.

The team of doctors on the case weren't sure of the relatedness of the Cancer to her previous breast cancer and they were also unsure of the relatedness of the Cancer to the Tamoxifen because of the type of Cancer it was.

What they did know was that my mom's Cancer was aggressive and undifferentiated, which means very hard to treat and that it had already broken out of the cervical cavity.

The Oncologist recommended six five hour treatments of Chemotherapy and that was Carboplatin and Paclitaxel which are highly toxic and very powerful drugs.

However, he was not at all optimistic about the results of the treatment and he added that with or without chemotherapy, life expectancy in such cases was a matter of months.

My siblings and I decided not to inform my mom of the statistics and let her make the decision of just how she felt and she opted for treatment.

She saw that her only option at that point because there were no other alternatives offered by the doctors. It was either Chemotherapy or nothing so she said okay, lets' do it.

On March 18, six weeks after surgery, Chemotherapy began and within a week, my mother was in the emergency room.

That was in the week of the first treatment, she had to be treated for Pleural Effusion. Now the Pleural lining is the lining around the lung and it was filled with fluid and she was hardly able to walk.

She could do nothing without breathing very heavily and the doctors were very concerned so they had to bring her into the emergency room.

They pulled out quarts of fluid from her lungs. In fact, hers was the second largest amount of fluid on record at _____ Hospital at the time.

And when they did the biopsy of the fluid, the report read positive for malignancy, Papillary Adenocarcinoma consistent with Metastasis from patients known Papillary Serous Adenocarcinoma of the Endometrium, which means, in short, it had spread to the lining of her lungs.

So, it was from the Peritoneal wall into the lung lining so, it was not a good sign. Over the next week, her condition just worsened.

Her weekly blood test revealed a very low Hemoglobin count.

It went down to 8.6 and on March 31st, she was brought in for blood transfusion.

And although all of these treatments are helpful and were keeping her alive, they were having terrible effects themselves on my mother.

She has a bit of fear of open places and strange people and it was all overwhelming to her.

And just even the physical treatment itself was frightening and disturbing other symptoms and systems in her body.

Her bowel was impacted and her urinary problems began, It had been on-going but they intensified and then she developed an infection, which was very frightening.

She was put on antibiotics and thankfully they worked but the antibiotics have side effects.

The doctor considered stopping the treatment because the treatments were killing my mother, in addition to the disease.

Right before the next treatment, my mom showed some improvements.

She felt a little better and so she talked to the doctor and decided to continue and he said, well, if she wants to, okay, although he was not really in favor of it.

Soon afterwards, her bowel infection worsened and with her urination increasing in frequency, she was no longer able to walk to the bathroom.

So, it was very messy. It was very problematic. It was a major concern.

So, they took a blood glucose test and that revealed a 600 blood sugar level, which was not good at all so, my mom was placed immediately on Insulin.

Too many things had gone wrong with my mother's health and the family, we were falling apart. We were having a great deal of difficulty of holding together.

Mike-

Wow.

What did you do?

Dr. Pat-

Well, I think personally what I did was resisting the spiraling downward, this great despair that we were locked into and unable to get out of.

I have been connected with Medical Mission Sisters over the years and, I've not gone there a few years but a friend of mine was visiting and brought me over.

And I was introduced about a year prior to what just happened to my mom. I was introduced to all the new holistic health techniques that they were offering and I remembered that, I remembered that and I thought that it's worth a shot.

I went over and I talked to the Sisters and if they could help. I explained my mom's condition and asked if there was anything available, anyone available and that there would be a need for the person to come to my house because my mom is too sick to get up.

And, they said they would ask to see if someone has the time to do that.

And they would talk to the Sisters there and a few weeks later, I got a call from Sister Yumiko.

And she's willing to come out and she came to talk to us.

And she said that she would begin Reiki.

So on May the 19th, Sister Yumiko came to our home and began Reiki on my mom. And my mom is a very unsophisticated person as she's not educated.

She doesn't get out of her home much. She knows basically her family and not much beyond that so she had no idea of what Reiki was or anything about alternative healing techniques.

But she was open to try and there were certain circumstances about it that made it good.

First of all, this woman was willing to come to our home.

So, my mom didn't have to be bombarded by hospitals and scary people, and scary things entering her body.

And also, when she met Sister Yumiko, she was so pleased by the peace, profound peace that sister brought.

I get a little emotional.

Mike-

Giggle...

Dr. Pat-

She just brought beautiful peace and hope.

Mike-

That's what Sister Yumiko does.

Dr. Pat-

Yeah

Uh, now, the immediate effect on my mother was very strange.

Sister Yumiko warned us ahead of time.

She said it might. She concentrated on her bowel because that was the major problem at the time.

My mom was so impacted and the doctors were doing nothing about it.

She's had terrible stuff, stomach pains and she just was going from severe constipation to severe diarrhea.

So Yumiko focused on her stomach as the first problem...that was the worst at the time.

And she warned us ahead that there might be increased activity and discomfort and that we could call her in case that should happen.

She felt lots of activity.

She would talk to my mom

You know, she talked to my mother, did the session and my mother didn't ask me any questions because she didn't even know what to ask.

But, uh, I noticed a few days after the first session...immediately after and for a few days, there was increased bowel activity and discomfort.

I didn't call Sister Yumiko.

I just waited and watched to see what happened.

I trusted the process, I trusted the Sister, I trusted what was happening between the Sister and my mother.

Even though it was scary at first to see the increased activity, I thought it would go well.

It seemed it would go well.

And in the first few days, it did sort of die down and I saw that the increased discomfort was relieved.

So Sister came the second time, that following Wednesday.

And the immediate effect was positive this time.

As soon as the Sister finished the Reiki, my mother sat up and she asked for something to eat.

And this is remarkable because one of the worst effects of the Cancer was my mom had lost her appetite.

The first six months prior actually to the surgery, she stopped eating and had lost so much weight.

And food is no longer interesting to her.

And for an Italian woman she knows that she no longer was able to not only generate interest in food for herself but she could no longer supply food for her family and that's her life.

So, the kitchen and food, that was a big deal for her.

The simple statement that I'm hungry, what do we have to eat?

My hair, I felt it was standing straight on top of my head.

That was, like, so remarkable.

From just a simple sentence, it was so remarkable.

My mother would now be hungry.

So, I flew into the kitchen.

And got her something to eat and delighted in that.

That was the first sign.

Then, she asked to watch television.

And that was her first interest in television since the surgery.

I saw that as very positive.

And that happened each time Yumiko came.

She came weekly.

Now, the first she came for an hour.

But after seeing my mom, she realized that 60 minutes was too much for my mother.

You know, for other people, I am sure an hour was fine.

But my mom, like I said, is unsophisticated.

And just to even lie quietly for 60 minutes was a big deal.

So, Yumiko was very willing to try whatever would work and very open to try.

She said, lets' do 30 minutes.

So, she came weekly for 30 minute sessions.

And each week, my mom continued to improve until on June 23rd, they performed another CAT scan.

And that revealed no evidence of Cancer.

Mike-

Wow, wow, wow

She had started this treatment about May 19th?

Dr. Pat-

May 19th, yes.

Mike-

And this is June 23rd.

This is only what?

Five treatments?

Dr. Pat-

Five treatments, yes

Five treatments

Mike-

So, she went from totally bedfast and disinterested, and critical almost to...

Dr. Pat-

Yea, yea, yea total system breakdown

And with one system after the next breaking down from both the Cancer and the treatment. She lost interest, you know.

Mike-

That's a remarkable result within short period of time.

Dr. Pat-

Yes, yes and the...

In fact I was on retreat at the time that my mom went for the CAT scan.

I had gone away. It was very intense at home and I went away for a few days and my brother was taking care of my mother.

He took off a few days from work and he stayed with her.

And while I was on retreat, I had the distance and the time to reflect on the changes.

The incredible and miraculous changes that have been taking place and I could see all the good that was coming from this Reiki treatment.

During this time, this quiet time, this hopeful time, this healing time something came over me and I felt so sure that when I would go home, I would find that the CAT scan is going to be good.

That the results of that CAT scan were going to be good and I had the sense that there was no longer a problem.

I know, that was very strange and it was sort of going out on a limb to go that far to say that there was no problem.

But I felt in my heart that was the case before the last day. Before I left the retreat, I gave thanks.

And when I came home, I knocked on the door and my brother opened the door and he said I have news for you, from the CAT scan.

I said wait, let me pull my journal out and Let me read you the news Frank and I read it.

I said mom is healed, isn't she. It says it right here.

He said, how did you know?

He said the CAT scan revealed no evidence of cancer.

Not that she's getting better, not that the tumor had shrunk.

But that there was no evidence of Cancer in her body.

I flew out and I got a copy.

I went to the doctor and I got a copy of the report.

So, I had it in my hand and that it said no evidence of Cancer.

So, the Oncologist, at first he wanted to stop the Chemotherapy at that point which was only four of the six prescribed treatment.

He wanted to stop the Chemotherapy for two reasons

One because of the hopeful sign that there was no evidence of Cancer but also because my mom had developed a Neuropathy from the treatments, which means she was not able to walk.

You know, she would fall over constantly so, he thought that was very detrimental and she needed a break from the chemo.

But he intended to restart her on the chemo in a few weeks as soon as the Neuropathy had passed.

You know, he wasn't, I guess, as trusting of the results because the prognosis had been so negative in her case.

And I asked him if it was possible to stop the chemo.

Because my mom and I, you know, we were ready to stop at that point.

At least I was ready to stop.

I think, you know, I think we could stop at this point.

But he was not ready to stop because he said, no, in these cases we always give the six treatments.

I thought - You know, it's not going to work anyway but we have to give her everything that she can get and we went with that.

And then, when we went back in a few weeks for him to recheck her Neuropathy had improved, which should have been when she would go back on chemo.

And she was scheduled for the chemo.

He said no, no Chemotherapy.

And we were, like, wow.

We had brought sandwiches because it's a five hour treatment where she is strapped to that machine and receiving toxins in to her system for five hours, which was unbelievable. It was an incredible experience for her to go through so, we were ready, you know, tapes and everything to get through the experience. We didn't eat that lunch. We went out to Eat. We were so amazed that was the end of the Chemotherapy.

And it was, like, I felt dizzy. My head was so light, her head was so light. After we eat, we came home and just called everyone we knew.

My mom didn't have to go through that anymore, In fact, my mom, you know, just, what can I say, she was just delighted.

Mike-

Wow

Since you wrote the case history, it's been a month or more than a month, so what has been happening lately?

Dr. Pat-

She continued to show steady improvement.

In fact, we just called the Oncologist this week and she got another clean bill of health.

They keep a close eye on her.

Every three months, she either see s the surgeon or the Oncologist and gets another clean bill of health.

She no longer needs the walker or a cane.

She has begun to gain weight.

She showers a little.

She cooks. My mom now cooks.

She cooks for me, she cooks for herself, she cooks for her grandchildren. She cleans the house.

Her hair is fully grown.

She returned to her normal life.

She looks beautiful.

Her color has returned.

She has been taken off of just about all her medications.

The only thing that she takes now is digoxin for her heart and they lowered the medication for that.

Even her heart has improved and her heart was not indicated in the Cancer but her heart has improved.

She takes one little medication a day for her blood sugar and my guess is she doesn't need that.

There will probably be a point where they will even pull her off of that.

But other than that she just takes her vitamins. So there's no evidence of the return of the Cancer at this point and she's getting better on all fronts.

Mike-

How's her weight?

Dr. Pat-

It's good.

She had been 166 when all these problem started.

Then, she went down to 142.

And now, she's back up to 153.

Mike-

Great.

Dr. Pat-

Yes.

Mike-

What did the doctors and the Oncologist say about all this?

Dr. Pat-

Well, to use their words, they both used the same words.

They said it's remarkable.

They smiled.

The Oncologist never smiled.

Mike-

Laugh.

Dr. Pat-

He was always, like, sitting at the desk and he never cracked a smile once.

And then when her CAT scan, the June 26th CAT scan came back, he began smiling and he has used the word remarkable numerous times since and so has the surgeon. It was really unexpected.

Mike-

So, what does Dr. Pat think about this whole recovery?

What made the difference?

Dr. Pat-

Well, it's very clear to me.

In my opinion, it was the introduction of Reiki as well as Sister Yumiko's loving and peaceful presence that brought about this hope and this openness to a positive life force.

Rather than this spiraling death force that has taken us down and it was that movement with God's spirit and this incredible shedding off light, the Christ's light, the light of our faith on and through Sister into my mother and into the family, which is so devoted to each other and to move that devotion into a working together for the good and for life rather than for you know, just fighting the inevitability of death but to move into hope and life that brought about my mom's healing.

Mike-

Well Dr. Pat, I am very appreciative of your time.

I consider this presentation that you're sharing in to be a tribute to your mother. I consider it to be a gift in honor of Sister Yumiko, and her wonderful gifts that she gives to everybody that she meets.

And I think it is a gift to everyone that hears or reads these words because they can know that God is listening to their prayers.

And God is open to sharing healing with them and to bring the most wonderful gift to them if the will invite spirit in.

And Dr. Pat you have been a tremendous vehicle to share this blessing, share the blessing that your mother receives with so many other people that can share similar blessings with those that they love and care about .and I want to thank you so very much.

Dr. Pat-

Thank you very much and thank you for bringing so much hope into the world.

Mike

My pleasure.

I trust these stories have given you some ideas of what you can do for yourself and those you care about.

I invite you to celebrate life in all its variety at every opportunity.

**May all who read these words be Blessed
and may they be a blessing to all those that they love
AND SO IT IS!**

Resource List

Distant Healing Sessions –
  Physical Healing
http://LetMeHelpYouHeal.withMike.com
  Angel Healing
http://AngelHealing.withmike.com/

Other Books by Rev. Mike at www.Amazon.com–
Trauma Healing options for VA Hospitals: Help for Veterans to Own Their Healing and their
  future.
Trauma Healing Action Steps For Veterans: Help To Stat Healing
Trauma Healing Action Steps For Veterans: Empowerment
Trauma Healing Action Steps For Veterans: Forgiveness
Trauma Healing Action Steps For Veterans: Thought Freedom
Stress Release Energy Work: How To Cope
Angel Raphael Speaks Volume One: Take Courage! God Has Healing in Store for You
Angel Raphael Speaks Volume Two: Take Courage! God Has Healing in Store for You
Reiki Journaling From Japan
Reiki Is Alive: God's Great Gift
Four Parts To Healing
Distant Healing: We Are All Connected

Free Resources

Learn to dump fear at
http://TheGreatAmericanFearDump.withMike.com
Spiritually Prepare for Surgery
http://PrepareForSurgery.withRevMike.com

Angel Scribe messages at
http://www.SpiritualComfortCare.com
Law of Attraction Expert column at
http://www.ReverendMikeWanner.com
Stress Release at
http://www.StressReleaseCoach.com

Angel Raphael Speaks through Rev. Mike Wanner. I have channeled multiple message sets and they all have to be polished to smooth out my errors and negotiate some words that may be too easily misunderstood. Grammar is not polished as it is too easy to miss the subtlety of the energy flow. To find out the availability of messages and latest updates go to. http://www.spiritualcomfortcare.com/angel-raphael-speaks/

Also "Tell Mike your concerns – If he and I agree there is a broader need, messages may follow. Citizens of all nations invited as long as your write in English. Do not expect him to answer as he is very busy already listening to us." E-mail Mike at mikewann@voicenet.com.

May All Who Read This Be Blessed Reverend Mike Wanner
www.ReveredMikeWanner.com
www.AngelRaphaelSpeaks.com
www.StressReleaseCoach.com

Private Channeling

Angel Raphael Speaks is a series of free messages that are channeled through Reverend Mike Wanner for the Highest good and Highest Healing of all concerned.

Many questions arise about Reverend Mike doing private channeling and he does help with that at his site http://AngelHealing.withMike.com

Reverend Mike is available world-wide as a psychic channel, emotional release facilitator, spiritual energy practitioner & teacher, and public speaker.

He looks forward to meeting you soon!

Email - mikewann@voicenet.com 215-342-1270
http://AngelHealing.withMike.com

PRIVATE SPIRITUAL READINGS/channelings or Spiritual Healing Sessions: Telephone or in person

Rev. Mike is available for private, one-on-one intuitive sessions with you, his Guide Family, and your Guides. He helps by offering clarity on emotional situations about your life, your purpose, your spirituality, and the release of stuffed emotions and cellular memory.

Connect to the love of your Guides today! Contact Rev. Mike for an appointment.

Click on this link to go to the page –
http://AngelHealing.withMike.com

Sessions available:

1. Spiritual Readings

2. Angel Channeling
3. Distant Reiki Healing
4. Distant Clearing of Stuffed Emotions
5. Distant Clearing of Cellular Memory
6. Distant Clearing of Energy Blockages
7. Distant Clearing of the Chakras
8. Mastermind dowsing responses to yes/no direction finding questions.
9. Customized needs

Rev. Mike is a facilitator of healing. He brings you and the Divine together so that you can align with the Divine and have a great time and a great life. All healing is between you and God, as it should be.

Rev. Michael Wanner

Rev. Michael Wanner started his metaphysical and ministerial studies with Reiki in 1993 and has studied seven styles of Reiki in the U.S., Japan, Canada, Denmark and Australia. He is certified to teach. He became certified to teach Integrated Energy Therapy in 1999 and co-taught the first IET class of the new Millennium. Mike began dowsing in 2001.

Ordained as a Metaphysical Minister of the International Metaphysical Ministry and an Interfaith Minister of the Circle of Miracles Ministry, Rev. Mike practices and teaches spiritual energy therapies in the Philadelphia Area.

Rev. Mike holds ministerial degrees from the University of Metaphysics and the University of Sedona. He is a Pastoral Care Associate of Aria – Frankford Hospital. He taught at the National Academy of Massage Therapy and Health Sciences.

Rev. Mike was a faculty member of the Medical Mission Sister's Center for Human Integration's School of Integrated Body/Mind Therapies in Fox Chase, Philadelphia, PA for twelve years.

Rev. Mike is licensed by the teaching of Intuitional Metaphysics to practice Spiritual Healing and Scientific Prayer. Mike is also a Prayer therapist.

Rev. Mike was elected in 2007 to the status of "Fellow of the American Institute of Stress."

In 2008, Rev. Mike became a practitioner of Coincidental Recognition as he incorporated the CoRe system in to his spiritual healing practice.

In 2009, Rev. Mike trademarked a new healing process called Quantum Quatro! Subtle Energy System Support®.

In 2011, Rev. Mike joined the outreach program known as the Health Advantage Group.

In 2012. Rev. Mike became a Certified Professional Coach by The Master Coaching Academy and Joined The Personal Empowerment Group .

Prior to his metaphysical, ministerial and coaching studies, Rev. Mike worked for Sears Roebuck and Co. while in High School and after graduation until he joined the U. S. Air Force in 1965. He returned to Sears from Vietnam in 1969 and stayed until 1978. His final Sears assignment was as an efficiency expert in Methods - Operational Research and Development.

Rev. Mike volunteered with Burholme Emergency Medical Services from 1969 and is still a Life Member and Board of Directors Member. He started a private ambulance company in 1975 and worked professionally in the field until 2001 when he devoted his full attention to real estate investing, healing and coaching.